Skin

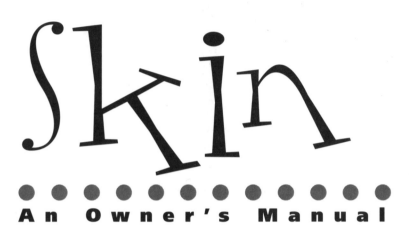

An Owner's Manual

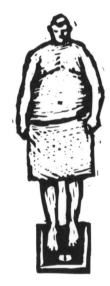

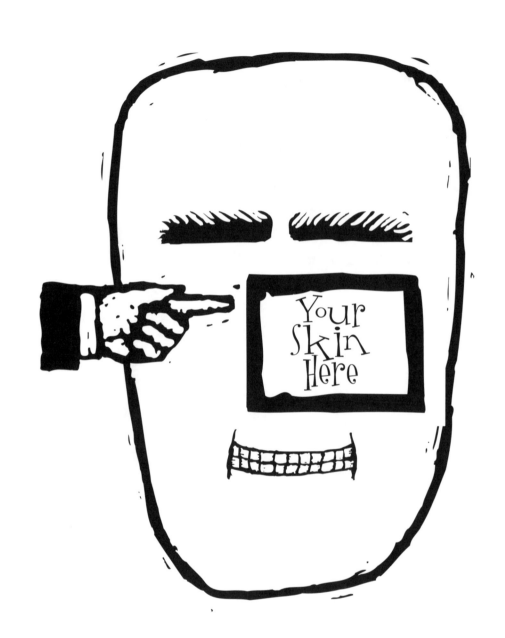

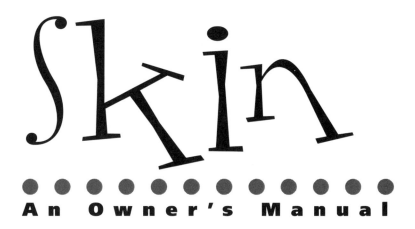

Skin

An Owner's Manual

What Your Skin Does for You
&
What You Need to Do for It

ROBERT BUCKMAN, M.D.

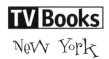

New York

PUBLISHER'S CATALOGING-IN-PUBLICATION
Buckman, Robert.
Skin : an owner's manual : what your skin does for you and what you need to do for it / Robert Buckman. — 1st ed.
p. cm.
Includes index.
ISBN: 1-57500-082-2
1. Skin—Care and hygiene. 2. Skin—Diseases—Popular works. 3. Dermatology—Popular works. I. Title.
RL87.B82 1999   612.7'9
        QBI99-944

Acknowledgments for permissions and credits for photographs appear on pages 102–103

The publisher has made every effort to secure permission to reproduce copyrighted material and would like to apologize should there have been any errors or omissions.

TV Books, L.L.C.
1619 Broadway, Ninth Floor
New York, NY 10019
www.tvbooks.com
Printed in Canada

a daly design

Contents

Introduction:

The Bare Facts

Viewed against the vast backdrop of the history of life on earth—from the first blob of living protoplasm in the primordial sea, right up to today when slightly more complex blobs of the same material call themselves politicians and run the whole show—skin is a fairly recent invention.

Before living organisms on earth evolved skin for themselves, they used a more primitive arrangement that is known to scientists as "skinlessness." Even today skinlessness is not extinct; it is the form of external covering currently favored by many primitive life-forms, including single-celled organisms, crustacea, and arachnids.

But human skin has evolved into a wonderfully complex and multi-functional organ. It regulates our interior environment, keeping our bodies at, well, body temperature whatever the outside temperature, humidity, or weather, and it bravely copes with a torrent of daily bangs, knocks, scrapes, cuts, and scuffs. In addition, our skin receives constant information about the state of the world outside and passes it on to us, while simultaneously transmitting signals about the state of our world-inside to any passing life-forms that may be interested. And it does all this with remarkably little fuss, going wrong only rarely.

This book will tell you how skin evolved to do all that, and how it manages to keep on doing it all day after day. You'll learn not only what our skin does for us, but also what we should be doing for it—and how we can help it to keep on doing its job.

Just one disclaimer before we start. This book isn't intended to be a comprehensive encyclopedia of skin and skin-care. It won't provide you with a complete dictionary of everything that can go wrong with your skin. What it will do is to give you an overview of the subject, focusing on the most interesting bits and leaving out the boring stuff. By the time you've finished this book, you will have acquired a serviceable understanding of how human skin performs its various functions, together with several extraordinary insights and dozens of reliable and useful tips.

1

Skin— Can't Leave Home Without It

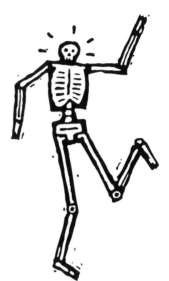

Your Inner Child and How to Keep It In

Before skin, there was skinlessness. Although that wasn't much of a problem in and of itself, it did impose a few limitations on life-forms. Without some form of wrapping, an animal couldn't go anywhere.

That may not make sense when you first think about it, but try this mental exercise. Imagine for a moment what life would be like if you were a simple single-celled organism swimming about in the primordial sea. (Oh, come on, just *try* and imagine it—it'll only take a moment and you won't feel a thing, honest.)

That's good, thank you.

Now, if you happen to be a type of organism called a paramecium then you probably look a bit like this

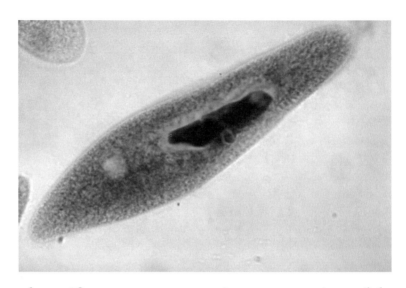

photo. If you are a paramecium you consist—solely and entirely—of one single cell, and your height is approximately a hundredth of the width of a human hair (even when you're standing up straight). All of your activities and functions—everything that you do—goes on inside that single cell of which you are composed. It's a bit like a one-room apartment in a big city. Your single room serves all your needs—it's your kitchen, dining room, living room, and bedroom. So, various specialized parts (organelles) of your single cell serve as food-processor, oven, dining table, toilet, ventilation, power-supply, central heating, bed, and so on. (This being the inside of a single cell, you don't get cable TV.)

So there you are, swimming in a very pleasant piece of primordial sea that happens to contain just the right amount of salt and oxygen, plus a bit of carbon dioxide, and a smattering of ammonia and a few other useful molecules.

As long as you're in that particular and pleasant bit of sea, everything is absolutely fine. You can take in the oxygen and the small molecules that you need through the wall of your single cell and you can gently and quietly excrete your waste product chemicals into the sea through the same wall. (And since you are very small you aren't even polluting the environment to any appreciable extent.)

Your only problem is that you can't go anywhere.

You are totally dependent on your external environment, which has to be absolutely perfect. If the sea around you gets saltier (if you're in a rock-pool that partly evaporates, for example) you will shrivel up like a raisin and die. If the water becomes less salty, you will expand like an over-inflated tire, explode, and die. If there's no oxygen or other essential molecules in the water around you, you will asphyxiate or starve—either way, you will die. If your children and grandchildren and the billions of descendants that you can create in a few months or so don't find somewhere new to live, their excretory products will eventually poison the water—there goes the neighborhood—and you will die.

Your existence may be fun but it is precarious.

If you want to travel, you've got to evolve a wrapper, something that will keep the inside of you warm and comfortable and balanced in terms of water and salt, and so forth no matter what the environment outside is like. You need a skin.

As the great French biologist Claude Bernard once put it, *"la fixitée du milieu interieur est la condition de la vie libre"* (roughly translated, it means: "if you can keep your insides steady and comfortable, you can go anywhere you like"). Obviously Claude Bernard's words echoed backward through five billion years of evolution, because that's exactly what life on this planet did. It decided to evolve skin and forage about, traveling everywhere, colonizing the planet, endangering the rain forests, and sending real-estate prices through the roof.

And it was the evolution of a packaging system that made all this possible.

Once animals managed to come up with a protective wrapping system—culminating in the evolution of skin—they could start moving about, exploring new environments and surviving a whole range of external environmental conditions (or in English, weather). To put it in a nutshell, the protective wrapping around animal life forms evolved in order to keep the outside world out and the animal life form snug and cozy inside. As the animal life-forms on this planet became more complex, they evolved (roughly speaking) two forms of wrapping systems. One branch of the life-stream evolved its wrapping and skeletal support systems on the *outside*—this became what we now call an exoskeleton. Animals with an exoskeleton are quite hard and crunchy on the outside (think of a cockroach) and can keep their soft inner parts well protected inside their exoskeleton armor. (Until you step on them, that is.) The muscles they need to move their limbs and the plated body parts are attached to the inside of the exoskeleton. Examples of animals using this type of wrapping are the arthropods, which include the insects, ticks, and mites as well as lobsters, roaches, and spiders.

But the exoskeleton was only one possible solution to the wrapping problem. Other animal life forms chose a different direction: they evolved their skeleton *inside* the body (the endoskeleton). During the aeons required to evolve that, they needed a tough and resistant wrapping layer on the outside. It was time for skin.

Here's an overview of how the endoskeleton type of animal is designed. The muscles that move the skeleton are attached to the bones. The internal organs required to keep the animal supplied with oxygen and food and to take away waste products (i.e., the lungs, heart, kidneys, and all the other viscera that we evolutionary biologists call "offal") are partially protected inside bony cages (the ribcage and the pelvis). Which is well and good, except that if that were all there was, the resulting animal would have all the survival advantage in a predatory world of a spoonful of gelatin. If you've got your muscles and your giblets all arranged around your bones or partly nestled inside bony cages, they need to be properly protected. What is needed is an intelligent wrapper— a tough and flexible system that can protect the innards and the muscles and so on from casual harm caused by such external destructive forces as wind, heat, snow, hair-dryers, falling off your bike, assault with a blunt instrument, etc. The whole assembly required (if you'll forgive the teleological reasoning) a tough and self-renewing casing. And that's just what evolved. The endoskeleton branch of the animal kingdom evolved a specialized organ which covered all of the others, which was tough and scuff-resistant, and which could repair itself. Evolution might have produced woven nylon, which does all of those things (and if *that* had happened we'd all look like travel luggage and wouldn't be able to recognize each other at airport carousels), but it didn't. Evolution instead produced skin.

Skin is basically a multi-layered organ that grows from the bottom (the inside), and in which the cells get tougher and harder as they grow up and move towards the top (the outside).

The Self-Renewing Wrapper

The entire raison d'être of skin is, as we've seen, to keep the animal inside and the world outside, and this diagram shows you how those two basic functions are served by the fundamental structure of skin. The secret to the whole thing consists of two main design concepts: (a) the cells at the bottom of the skin divide and produce new ones, and (b) as the cells mature they produce a substance called **keratin** which makes them tough.

Keratin is one of the most

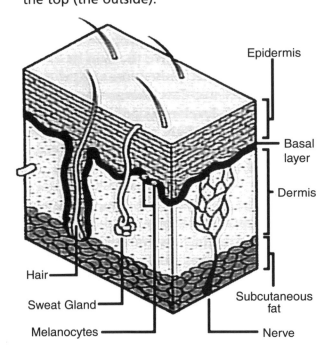

Epidermis

Basal layer

Dermis

Hair

Sweat Gland

Melanocytes

Subcutaneous fat

Nerve

amazing substances that has ever evolved. Its usefulness in animal biology puts it in the first rank alongside other astonishing evolutionary advances such as hemoglobin, DNA, mucus, Velcro, Teflon, and shampoo with built-in conditioner.

Keratin is a protein that has the extraordinary property of being tough and yet flexible. It's what makes skin so tough and scuff resistant. (Actually it's the elastin and collagen in the deeper layers that make the skin so leathery. Which means they also make leather so leathery.) Anyway, keratin is like a magically tough latex covering on the skin. When hairs become stuck together and super-soaked and matted in keratin, they turn into horns. The rhinoceros's horn, for example, is nothing but hair that has been matted together in a thick messy mass of keratin. (And you thought you had bad hair-days.) In less extreme moments, keratin makes our fingernails tough and smooth. Of course, human beings require another complex molecule called nail polish to provide colors that we can vary, which is why the forces of evolution have produced over 318,000 shades of this remarkable substance.

But, going back to keratin, it is not only a liquid form of armor, but it also happens to be toxic to cells when there's too much of it around. This means that as our skin cells grow up and mature, they fill up with keratin and then they die. Hence the toughest cells, on the outside of our skin, are all dead. This is lucky because it means we can lose them without suffering any pain (although the main reason we lose them painlessly is that there are no pain nerve endings in the outer layers). And as we shall discuss in chapter two, this means that we require a very subtle and adaptable control system that can match the number of cells being produced at the bottom layer to the number of cells being lost from the surface.

Wrap Music

So far, then, we've seen that the growth of skin cells is organized to provide a self-renewing system and that the cells toughen and die as they fill with keratin. Those two design concepts are only a start. But before we go on with the other ways in which skin meets animals' needs, I need to explain the simplistic way in which I'm using the word "evolution" and why it's not the actual way things work.

To make all this easier to understand, I'm going to continue to explain the development of skin as if evolution was some kind of Celestial Designer, shaping everything to fit the needs of the animal.Of course, that's not the way evolution actually works.

Evolution works—as we're all taught in school—by the process of natural selection, which is basically blind. It does not work towards any Final Concept or Ultimate Design for the finished product. There is no such thing. It leads to "improvement" when something new is produced that has some sort of advantage over what is there already. Let me explain.

Let's take the example of the evolution of keratinized skin. What happens is that one day an animal is born with slightly tougher and hornier skin due to keratin. That animal has a survival advantage and breeds more successfully than its softer-skinned, more vulnerable peers, so it dominates the herd and gets to pass its genes on to likewise tougher children. Actually, the same sort of process goes in most government departments and in many multi-national corporations nowadays—the thickest-skinned and toughest members of the brood survive, though of course in those corporate settings we don't call it "natural selection" we call it "economic right-sizing."

Anyway, for the purposes of this book, I'm going to talk as if natural selection knew what it wanted in the end. In real life, it doesn't—it just produces a well-adapted species by killing off the less-useful mutants.

Other Ingredients Include: Oil and Sweat (Some Restrictions Apply)

A skin that is tough and self-renewing still needs to be flexible and waterproof. Furthermore, it needs to let the animal keep cool in hot weather.

The flexibility and waterproofing is mostly done by a chemical mixture called sebum. Sebum is a thick, oily fluid that is made in special glands called sebaceous glands which are found clustered around the

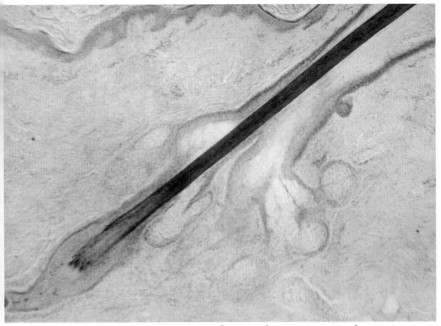

base of hair follicles. They make the sebum and squirt it out onto the surface of the skin around the shaft of the hair. It is thought that the sebum originally provided a major advantage in effective waterproofing, and it oils and lubricates the skin at the same time.

Hair-root and sebaceous gland

In fact, when we say that someone's skin appears to be oily, it is not oil that causes that appearance, it's sebum. All in all, sebum is jolly good stuff and an important lubricant and water-repellant, although, as we'll see in chapter five, the glands that make it can quite easily become blocked, which is the start of acne.

So now our prototype skin is tough, flexible, and waterproof. But while it's been evolving as the outside of the animal, the animal has been busy evolving an enormously complex set of biological systems inside. Eventually these systems become so complex that they need to be kept at a constant temperature to keep running reliably (in the same way that old-fashioned computers would conk out if they were allowed to overheat).

Which is where **sweat** comes in.

Or rather comes out.

Sweat is a very useful substance—it's mostly water (with a little added salt and small amounts of some other substances including pheromones). The clever thing about sweat is that it evaporates from the surface of the skin, and as it does it cools the skin down. This is because of a physical phenomenon that we all had to learn about in our seventh grade science class called the latent heat of vaporization. To explain it simply, as a liquid evaporates into a vapor, it takes some heat from its surroundings. This is called latent heat, because as the liquid takes in that heat, it doesn't get warmer, it simply changes its form from liquid to gas. All liquids do this—sweat in particular.

During the evolution of the warm-blooded animal species, including the mammals, it seems likely that the Forces of Nature had to take Grade Seven Science, because they clearly knew all about the latent heat of evaporation, and invented sweat accordingly.

Sweat is produced by the logically named sweat glands which occur in most areas of the body, but which are particularly dense on (on bad days) the forehead and in the forested areas such as the armpits. The sweat glands not only make the sweat but can also squirt it out quite quickly onto the skin when external conditions demand it (e.g. when it's hot weather or when you're in court).

The primary objective of sweat is to cool

down the skin—and the infrastructure of the skin plays a very important part in that. Skin has far more than its fair share of blood vessels running through it. In fact, at any instant about one-fifth of the blood coming out of the body headed for all parts of the body ends up going through the skin. One fifth! The rest of the body (including your brain, bowels, kidneys, and assorted tripe) has to fight over the remaining 80 percent. According to some calculations, each square centimeter of skin contains about two hundred yards of blood vessels.

Why does skin get such a lion's share of the blood supply? Because of its importance in temperature regulation. That's why.

The point is that when the outside temperature rises and the body begins to overheat, the skin pumps out extra amounts of sweat. The extra sweat evaporates, and that cools down the skin. At the same time, the blood vessels in the skin open up and the 20 percent of the circulatory volume flows through the skin, getting nicely cooled down as it does so. It's a bit like the way a refrigerator works—you have a little pump-thingy that gets cold, and then the refrigerator pumps coolant through it and the coolant gets cold and can be pumped all round the inside walls of the refrigerator. The only difference between the human arrangement and the General Electric ditto is that we keep all our insides at body temperature, which would melt our popsicles and spoil our frozen peas.

This physiological adaptation to high temperature

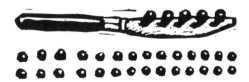

can be recognized by interested observers because: (A) the skin—and hence the person—goes red due to the increased blood flow through the skin and (B) the increased sweat production creates further visible changes such as deep stains in the underarm areas of the clothing, described by social scientists such as Tom Wolfe as "saddlebags." These, in turn, may cause further reddening of the face, depending on who's looking.

To be slightly more serious for a moment, there are some very interesting features of sweating which show that it is quite a complex adaptive biological response.

As I said above, sweat contains a fair amount of salt, which doesn't matter very much in moderate temperatures. But when a human moves from a cool or a warm climate to a hot climate, he or she can run into severe biochemical problems caused by losing large amounts of salt in the sweat. In extreme cases, this may cause very severe muscle cramps and weakness. One way of preventing this, is for the person to take in more salt (either in the form of juices or by taking salt tablets). But the interesting thing is that after a few days, the body's system adapts itself. As the body's systems becomes heat-adapted, the person produces large amounts of sweat—which help keep the person cool—but the sweat contains markedly less salt. In other words, the body adapts to the hot climate by producing a larger volume of sweat which is more watery and less salty. Which is quite impressive, when you think about it.

So, when you find yourself in a hot climate, make sure you take in lots of salt in your first few days (fruit juices, Gatorade, and so on) and wear clothes that allow you to sweat profusely.

Sweaty Messages

There may be other signals in sweat, too. It has been known for many years that sweat carries chemicals called **pheromones** which are basically a chemical signaling system (an external version of the internal hormones, really, hence their name).

These signals are undetectable (they don't really have an odor that anyone could recognize or describe) but they do have effects. They may create attraction (like musk) or aggression or anxiety, and they are apparently implicated in the hysteria of crowds. For example, it is thought that pheromones produce behavioral and biochemical changes in teenagers at rock concerts.
They are also responsible 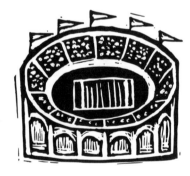 (so I'm told) for the exceptional attractiveness of certain singers at such concerts (a force which may be inexplicable by any other means, so far as the parents of the audience can tell). Pheromones are added to sweat in certain areas of the body, but not in others. If I remember correctly, the

pheromone-containing sweaty areas are called the **eccrine** areas, and the just-doing-my-job-cooling-the-body areas are called **apocrine** areas.

We are only just beginning to understand the complexities and power of pheromones. However, from what we know so far, they seem to be species-specific. This means that the pheromones that send signals of attraction from, say, one raccoon to another raccoon won't do a thing for, say, teenage humans at a rock concert. This (and I am extrapolating on a theme of my own here) may account for the fact that so few of the members of the audience at a rock concert are raccoons. Though perhaps it's merely that they can't afford the tickets. Or are tone-deaf (no, that can't be it, surely).

Anyway, it is often said that the musk secreted by certain female moths is a good model of a pheromone and can be detected by a male of the same species at a distance of over two miles. At this distance the final concentration of the scent is absolutely miniscule—one part per billions and billions of parts of air—yet the material is so powerful that is is detectable and virtually irresistible.

Anyway, that's pheromones, and they are an additional ingredient in sweat.

So far, then, we have seen what skin is meant to be doing and how its structure aids its function.

Now let's move on consider how skin controls its own growth and doesn't wear out or grow to be two feet thick.

2

A Growth Industry

Normal Growth

I'm going to start our discussion about the skin's growth rate with an astounding fact.

As I explained in the Introduction, skin cells grow from the bottom of the skin and as the cells migrate upwards they fill up with keratin, they die, and they are shed from the surface. This happens to literally millions and millions of cells per day. In fact—and you're not going to like this thought—most of the dust that accumulates in our houses is actually composed of dead skin cells. It has been calculated that over 90 percent of house dust is no more than (and no less than) dead and shed skin. So when you vacuum your carpet and your shelves and the couch and then you empty the vacuum cleaner it shouldn't surprise you that the stuff you empty out into the garbage can is a light gray color. It's always gray because that's what your skin looks like when it's in little bits. It's an odd thought that what you empty out of your vacuum-cleaner today was covering your leg yesterday. Oh dear, let's change the subject.

Mite Is Right

Be it ever so humble, the house dust that we create every day from our sell-by-date-expired skin cells is hearth and home to quite a few little critters. The

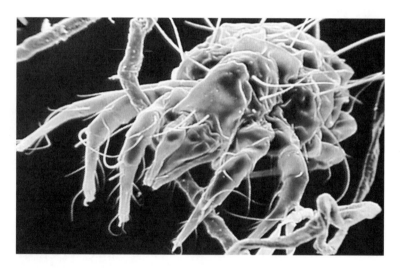

oddest of the skin-is-home-to-me gang is this little monster. His proper name is *Dermatophagoides pteronyssimus*, but you can call him by his nickname—the house dust mite. Actually, now that I come to think about it, the name of his genus is *pteronyssimus*, and the "p" is silent as in *psalm* (or, as they used to say in the old days, "the 'p' is silent as in swimming"). So you could, if you wished, call him Ptery for short, which would be pronounced Terri. This might start a whole new fashion in nicknames, e.g., Ptom, Ptim, Ptony, Ptina, Ptrish, Ptracy, Ptallulah, Ptarzan, etc.

Sorry, I got distracted.

Anyway, back to the realities of the dust mite and his ecology. Although they look like something out of *Star Wars* at this magnification, in fact dust mites are very small—only a few times the width of a human hair. The problem is that their bodies happen to include a whole bunch of proteins that are extremely irritating to the air passages inside certain people's lungs. As it happens, allergy to the dust mite is very common in people who have asthma, and exposure to a shower of dust mite protein (and droppings) can trigger or worsen an asthma attack in many people who are prone to them.

Which brings me on to a very useful hint.

If you happen to be asthmatic it's worth trying to reduce your exposure to house dust and (by implication) to the thousands of mites that call it home. It's worth making sure that your carpets and upholstery and shelves and flat surfaces are as dust-free as you can manage. Then make sure you change your socks or panty hose (which is where a lot of your shed skin cells will end up) every day. And— well worth an experiment, this one—try wrapping your mattress and your pillow in a polythene cover before you put the linen on. That way the amount of house dust- 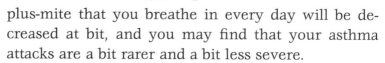 plus-mite that you breathe in every day will be decreased at bit, and you may find that your asthma attacks are a bit rarer and a bit less severe.

To give you some impression of how much skin you lose every day: it is said that it's almost the equivalent in weight of an average cigarette lighter (whatever they are). From the point of view of imagining the turnover rate of normal skin, that's a pretty impressive statistic. Since your skin under normal circumstances stays the same thickness and doesn't suddenly develop huge holes (unless you've been shot or something) this means one thing. Every day, your skin loses a cigarette-lighter's weight in cells, and each and every day your skin replaces the same number of cells by cell multiplication in the bottom layer.

This phenomenon is an example of a biological **dynamic equilibrium**—a genuinely wonderful phenomenon. Almost all biological systems in the world work on the same principle. We have a steady amount of blood in our veins because our red cells are manufactured by our bone marrow at the right rate to replace the number that wear out and are destroyed every day. The same is true of other high-traffic areas in our bodies—the linings of our mouths, stomachs, and bowels: all of these areas (like the skin) lose enormous numbers of cells every day, 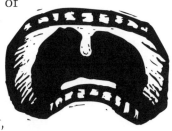 and replace them with new cells formed by cell multiplication at the same rate as the rate of loss. You can think of a dynamic equilibrium as being a bit like a high-volume bank account: the balance stays the same even though thousands of dollars worth of checks are written every day, because the same amount of money is paid in every day. (A state that I have always wanted to attain but have never managed.)

The exact mechanisms by which the human body controls this dynamic equilibrium in the skin is not yet fully understood. We know something about how it works in other areas—for example, in the way the bone marrow makes enough red blood cells. In that case, when the body starts running short of red cells the imminent deficiency is detected and a hormone called erythropoietin is manufactured (by the kidney, as it happens). Erythropoietin is a "speed-up" signal to the bone marrow, which is prodded into increased production and pushes out more red cells until the deficiency is made up.

A similar system exists for the skin, but we don't know all the components yet. Furthermore, it's all or-

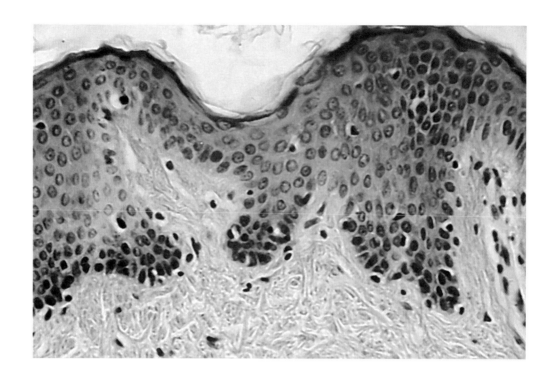

ganized locally (there doesn't seem to be a skin-equivalent of erythropoietin that circulates through the whole body). Somehow, an increased loss of skin cells (e.g. after an injury or a surgical incision) creates a local surge of chemical signals that we call growth factors. (We know the names of some of these: for instance, Epidermal Growth Factor or EGF for short.) These growth factors create a spurt of growth in the bottom layer of the skin and the deficiency is quickly made up.

Without getting too gee-whiz about this, it is quite extraordinary how quickly skin can repair itself. Think for a moment about what happens after surgery. The skin is completely cut, yet within a day the skin cells are going crazy repairing the defect. After two days they've already partially filled the gap, and by a week the scar is almost as strong as any other part of the skin.

But the really astonishing part is what happens next: when the defect is repaired, all that incredibly rapid growth and multiplication stops. I suppose it's like a space-shuttle—it flies a quarter of a million miles or so around the earth, and then lands and parks within two feet of where it's supposed to be.

The skin does the same thing. It speeds up its growth rate by a factor of thousands, and then when the job is done, it goes back to its normal rate.

Most of the time. Sometimes, it doesn't

Over-Enthusiasm in the Manufacturing Industry

Interestingly, in some people those mechanisms are not quite as accurate as in others. In some people, after a surgical incision, for example, the skin will go on growing a bit too long, producing a heaped-up or **hypertrophic** scar. (This isn't the fault of the surgeon, by the way, it's just the way some people's skin-growth control mechanisms are set.) In other people (more common in dark-skinned races than in light-skinned), a similar over-enthusiasm produces what are called **keloid** scars which have a rather glassy look to them and grow beyond the boundaries of the scar itself. Keloid scars—in the people who are prone to them—form more easily when the incisions are longitudinal (in the top-to-bottom direction) rather than when the incisions are side-to-side. We don't know why that is, but it is almost certainly related to the triggers that produce the growth factors in the skin and produce (or fail to produce) the "switch-off" signals when the repair is done. While we're on the subject, that glassy look to the scar is produced by excessive collagen manufactured by the fibroblasts, and sometimes injection of the scar with steroids is helpful in reducing the overgrowth.

In fact, a fault in that control system is probably the problem that underlies a fairly common skin condition, **psoriasis**. We don't fully understand how psoriasis is caused, but it probably has something to do with the failure of growth-control. What happens is that the skin goes into a mild over-production mode and keeps on producing extra skin cells which heap up and are shed from the surface in the form of those scaly patches. The scales that are shed from the surface are simply a sign that the skin is being a bit over-enthusiastic in its manufacturing habits. It's still a mystery as to why those patches are more likely to form on the outside of the elbows and front of the shins (rather than in the crook of the elbows and the back of the knees as happens with dermatitis or eczema). We assume that the growth-control system is partly inherited, because it seems that a tendency to develop to psoriasis runs in families. It's not easy to predict in the way the gene for eye-color is (if both your parents are blue-eyed, you'll be blue-eyed) but there is some genetic element in there somewhere.

Eventually, I predict, we'll know many more details about growth-control mechanisms in general and it is possible that one day we may be able to treat patches of psoriasis by giving a growth-control inhibitory factor which will simply reduce the over-production to normal levels. At the moment, that isn't possible, so the standard treatments includes the use of ultraviolet light of the type "A" exposure, combined with oral medications called psoralens. The combination of psoralens with UV "A" is called, logically enough, PUVA. There are a few variants of PUVA, including some methods of using ultraviolet "B" light. And sometimes the oral medications called retinoids—which I'll talk about later—are used. Another thing that's inter-

esting is that psoriasis is sometimes affected by sunlight and by stress. Presumably there are several triggers that come together to prod the skin into
over-production.

3

Don't Let the Sun Shine In

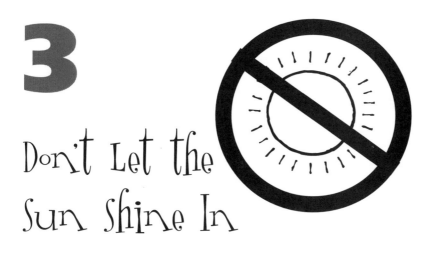

Melanin—Nature's Sunblock

So far, we have been discussing skin as a thoroughly wonderful and hard-working, self-renewing protectant against mechanical insults and the "thousand natural shocks that flesh would otherwise be heir to" (Shakespeare—almost). But in addition to the obvious physical dangers threatening the tenderest parts of the flesh, every animal under the sun is at considerable additional risk—from the sun itself. It's a bad-news-good-news story, really. The bad news is that the sun is basically a vast nuclear bomb giving off all kinds of destructive energy and environmentally harmful radiation and mess. The good news is that it's ninety-three million miles away (although it's a little

bit closer if you sunbathe on the roof of an apartment building rather than in the garden, of course). Anyway, by the time the sun's rays filter through the millions of miles of space and then through the earth's atmosphere, they contain more manageable amounts of energy. This is nice stuff if you can get it—and you can get it with the right kind of pigment. What you need is a pigment that can absorb some of the energy in sunlight and then turn that energy into a chemical dynamo for your cell's metabolism. Fortunately, there is such a pigment (if there wasn't, then life on this planet would never have evolved, and you wouldn't be reading this—for that matter I wouldn't have written it, either). Anyway, this light-entrapping pigment is called **chlorophyll**.

The only problem is that the world-wide franchise for chlorophyll was bought up by the plant kingdom and not by the animal kingdom. This means that animal life forms don't have any chlorophyll at all and are therefore incapable of directly utilizing the energy in the sun's light to produce useful chemicals. The animals solved this particular problem in a rather neat way: they decided to eat the plants. So, to put it simply, the plants spend all their time and effort turning sunlight into carbohydrates and protein and things, then the animals just breeze along and scarf up the proceeds. It's nature's version of capitalism.

OK. Now you understand that animal life requires the existence of sunlight so that plant life can use the sunlight to create fuel. The only snag with that is that sunlight just happens to be damaging to our skin. The ultra-violet portions of the sun's spectrum (notably the A and the B parts of the ultra-violet range) have the right kind of radiation to damage animal cells. There are actually two quite distinct ways in which sunlight can damage animals cells, by (a) genetic damage and (b) cooking it.

When you sunbathe what you do is cook your skin.

If you are pale-skinned and daft enough to sunbathe for many minutes without protection, you will see that your skin goes red (usually within minutes to hours), then may blister (in a few hours), and may even fall off (which, if it happens, is a Very Bad Sign Indeed). These are all simple effects of solar energy heating up the cells of your skin and killing them. However, those effects are not long-lasting and not really serious.

The other type of damage is potentially far more dangerous. Sunlight can cause damage to the genetic material—the DNA—of cells without actually killing them. Cells that have been damaged in this way may later go seriously wrong when they divide and reproduce. In fact, one of the most severe types of problems is that cells damaged in this way may produce cancers. We'll be talking about skin cancers in more detail in a moment, but just in case you feel deeply alarmed right now, let me tell you straight away that skin cancers are very common. The vast majority of them are of two types—the squamous cancers and the basal-cell cancers—neither of which ever spread to areas outside the skin, and are therefore not a threat to life. The third kind of skin cancer—melanoma—is much rarer, but, as we shall see, has the potential for spreading to distant areas of the body.

Fortunately, human skin contains its own protectant against sun-damage, a brownish pigment called **melanin**.

Melanin is nature's sunblock. It's a wonderful and serviceable pigment produced in the lower layers of the skin by cells called (logically enough) melanocytes. They produce the melanin, which is then taken up by the ordinary skin cells, the keratinocytes, which hold on to it. When the skin is exposed to lots of sunlight, the body accelerates the production of melanin by stimulation of a hormone called melatonin. When there is little sunlight, the body downsizes its melanin production and you end up looking pasty and white as if you lived in a cellar which, as we shall see, is generally a safer option.

As it happens, the skin can produce extra melanin in two ways. It can increase the general amount of melanin so that white skin steadily becomes more beige, and it can produce little splodges and blobs of melanin, which we call freckles, beauty spots, or moles (depending on what we think of them). I shall be discussing some of these briefly and in a very casual manner at the end of this chapter. Before that, let's talk about one of the most socially controversial issues around the distribution of melanin in human skin, namely the difference between what we call "black skin" and what we call "white skin."

Skin Color—You Won't Believe It Until You See It in Black and White

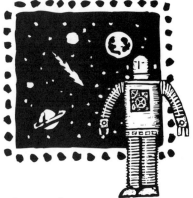

If you happened to live on the planet Mars and you happened to have specialized in comparative dermatology among life forms in the solar system, you would think that human beings on the planet Earth were stark staring bonkers.

As a Martian dermatologist, you would have absolutely no idea why human beings referred to some of their number as "black" and others of their number as "white." It would baffle you totally and cause to scratch one of your many heads in bewilderment. To you, humans would simply be slightly different shades of brown.

By contrast, to us earthlings this division of our species into dark-skinned races and light-skinned races is so embedded in our culture that we cannot,

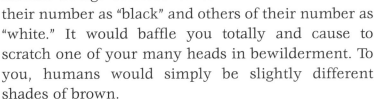

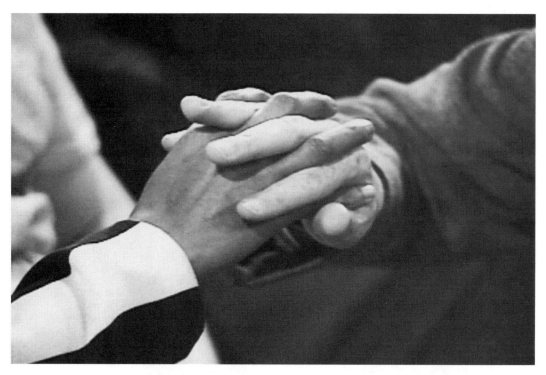

My hand interlaced with Julia's.

even for a moment, imagine any other way of looking at skin color.

But . . . it has virtually no basis in reality at all.

Look at this picture of my hand and Julia's hand.

We are so accustomed to seeing images like this that we would say "there are five white fingers interlaced with five black fingers." But from a dermatological point of view this is total and utter nonsense. Let me demonstrate by showing you photographs of black skin and of white skin as they appear under the microscope. In these pictures the melanin pigment appears as little dark-grey splodges near the bottom of the skin (in color photographs you would see them as a medium-brown color). Look at this photograph:

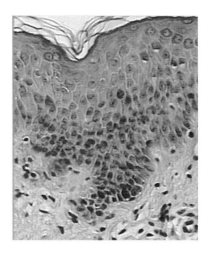

Photomicrograph of black skin

What you see here is the usual pattern of layers of skin cells, and towards the bottom of the skin you see a few splodges of melanin.

What is really surprising is that this picture is a specimen of what we call black skin.

Now while that picture is still fresh in your memory, look at the next picture. There's no difference, is there? What we call white skin has got exactly the

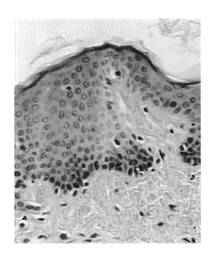

Photomicrograph of white skin

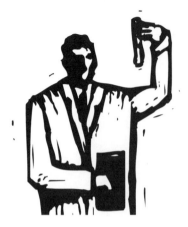

same amount of melanin as what we call black skin. In fact there is a difference, but it's so small that you would only be able to detect it at much greater magnification—under an electron microscope. When you look at skin cells using an electron microscope, you can see that in white skin the melanin inside the skin cells is bundled up in little packages. In black skin there is the same amount of melanin but it is spread out evenly throughout the whole skin cell. And that's it. That's the only difference there is.

Color is a simple matter of micro-packaging.

The old proverb goes "we're all the same color under the skin" but in fact it's even more true to say "we're all the same color even within the skin."

And if you were that dermatologist from Mars you might even be tempted to say after you'd seen those photographs: "It hardly seems worthwhile making a big fuss about such tiny differences." And you'd be right.

Get Real—Slip-Slop-Slap

Melanin, as we said, is nature's way of protecting the cells in the skin (and therefore the cells below) from sun damage. So dark-skinned human beings had a real natural selection advantage in parts of the world where there is lots of sun. In the temperate and polar regions, sun damage is much less of a problem, so the survival advantage of melanin was less and light-skinned races did just fine, thank you.

Until they started sunbathing, which happened when that became fashionable.

Which brings me to a very important point, namely the social significance of suntan.

In the Victorian era, the upper-crust of society (the lords and ladies) got very little exposure to sun. When they walked outside, they wore tons of clothing and used parasols and hats, hence their skin had very little exposure to sun. By contrast, manual laborers were out in the sun all day with their sleeves rolled up and so developed ruddy complexions and suntans. In the Victorian era, the elite did their darnedest to maintain a porcelain-white skin, and they regarded a suntan as a very low-class status symbol.

Things have changed.

For the last few decades, we have come to regard a suntan as a sign of someone who has enough money to take the leisure-time to bask in the sun. Far from being a symbol of incessant manual labor, it is now the symbol of moderate wealth and leisure, particularly in winter.

In Canada, where I live, the sort of people who strut around with a deep suntan in January are very clearly the sort of people who can afford a winter holiday in the Bahamas or in Florida. (Which prompts one to ask why they have bothered to come back to Canada in mid-winter. The answer is usually, "to gloat, of course.")

Suntan has therefore become a social statement—but it is NOT a health statement.

Skin that has been exposed to lots of sun is very likely to develop wrinkles, and is also at a higher risk of developing one of the types of skin cancer. This is particularly true if excessive exposure to sun has occurred when the occupant of the skin was young. In fact—to be quite serious for a moment—if a young person has had one or more blistering sunburns before the age of twenty, the risk of later developing the most dangerous form of skin cancer (melanoma) is increased five-fold. And five-fold is a lot.

Apart from smoking, then, sunburn is one of the most avoidable life-style cancer risks on the planet.

Let's take a moment and go over the main ways in which all of us can avoid major sun-damage to the skin (and still have fun). The secret here is to remember the catch-phrase "Slip-Slap-Slop" (this stands for these three basic rules: *slip* on a shirt, *slap* on a hat, and *slop* on the sun-block). To spell it out in greater detail, these things are really worth doing and they are all of particular importance for young children (i.e., up to late teens, at least):

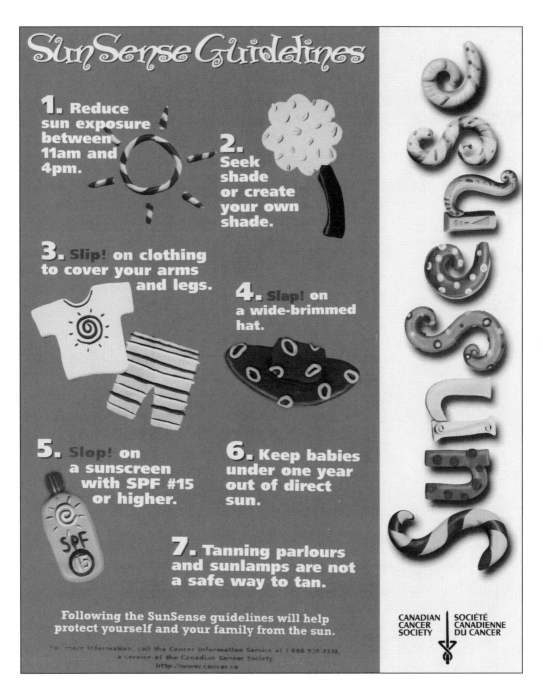

SunSense Guidelines

1. Reduce sun exposure between 11am and 4pm.

2. Seek shade or create your own shade.

3. Slip! on clothing to cover your arms and legs.

4. Slap! on a wide-brimmed hat.

5. Slop! on a sunscreen with SPF #15 or higher.

6. Keep babies under one year out of direct sun.

7. Tanning parlours and sunlamps are not a safe way to tan.

Following the SunSense guidelines will help protect yourself and your family from the sun.

For more information, call the Cancer Information Service at 1-888-939-3333, a service of the Canadian Cancer Society.
http://www.cancer.ca

CANADIAN CANCER SOCIETY | SOCIÉTÉ CANADIENNE DU CANCER

- Always wear a shirt or T-shirt when staying out-side in the sun, especially when swimming.

- Stay out of direct sunlight (e.g., in the shade or under an umbrella) for most of the time between 11 a.m. and 4 p.m.

- Wear a hat with a brim.

- Cover exposed skin with sunblock cream with a sun-protection factor (SPF) of at least 15.

- Reapply sunblock after swimming or after several hours (even the waterproof ones won't stay on indefinitely).

And, while we're on the subject, we don't know for certain that sun-tanning parlors are safe. In general, it's PROBABLY worth avoiding the risk. Although a mild suntan is probably not a significant hazard to your health, there's no evidence that continually tanning your skin, sometimes to a more-than-mild extent, is actually safe.

Sorry about that, but it's better to know the situation rather than take a risk (however small) without knowing it.

One Brief and Important Note—When to Think About a Melanoma

Even though this book is not intended to serve as a comprehensive or major dictionary of the ills that can afflict the skin, it's worth making a few genuine points about the rarest form of skin cancer, **melanoma**. So this section won't be funny, but it might be helpful.

Melanoma (often called malignant melanoma) is a very rare kind of skin cancer. The two common skin cancers (the squamous cell cancer and basal cell cancer) account for about 97 percent of all skin cancers and they are never a threat to life or health, although they can be a nuisance.

Melanoma is rare but it can be, in some cases, potentially dangerous since sometimes it can spread from the skin to other areas of the body.

Some melanomas develop in areas of skin that have not had any sun-damage, but a high proportion are partly caused severe sun-damage. This is one major reason why we need to take precautions about letting the sun damage skin. In fact, the risk of later developing a melanoma (as mentioned above) is increased five-fold if you suffer a blistering sunburn before you are twenty years old. Prevention of melanoma is the best form of treatment.

If a melanoma does develop, then early treatment is really important. If a melanoma is removed when it has not gone deeply into the skin, the chance of complete and permanent cure is very high indeed.

Hence any colored mole that might be a melanoma should be seen and assessed by a physician with expertise in the topic as soon as possible.

Moles are very common and melanomas are very rare, but you should ask a physician to assess any mole:

- If it has an irregular outline (as opposed to being small and circular).

- If it changes color or develops colorless areas inside it.

- If it develops other little moles around it.

- If it is growing or if it is bigger that about a quarter of an inch (the width of a pencil).

- If you are unsure about it or if you can't assess it easily (e.g. if it's on your back).

- If it bleeds when you touch it accidentally.

If you have lots of moles on your body, it may be worth asking your physician if you should have an assessment by a dermatologist so that you can be advised if any are suspicious.

One final point, which is an important and reassuring one: in many cases, it is impossible to be absolutely certain whether a mole is a simple mole or a melanoma. For that reason, biopsies are done—and rightly so!—for many moles that turn out to be, thank goodness, nothing serious at all. So, if your doctor recommends a biopsy don't panic. It does not necessarily mean that he or she thinks you have a melanoma. Usually it just means that one can't be certain the mole is innocent until it's been removed.

Beauty Spots & the Eye of the Beholder

So, melanin is the skin's own natural pigment which was originally designed to protect against sun damage. But melanin also occurs in discrete areas on the skin. We call some of these freckles and others beauty spots or moles (depending on whether we like the way they look or not). What has happened with pigmented moles is that they have come to carry some very strong socially-defined signals. As a society we have decided what it beautiful and what is not, and we've made it a big deal. Look at this example.

In the TV studio, we held an impromptu beauty competition. Disappointingly, I came second, but I must be honest, the woman who won—Lisa—did look a tad more like a beauty queen than I did. Anyway, I soon overcame any bitterness that I might have felt, and we did a simple demonstration concerning the positioning of localized melanin. In this photo, you will, I think, agree that Lisa looks extremely attractive. Her beauty spot (albeit manufactured from colored latex) is

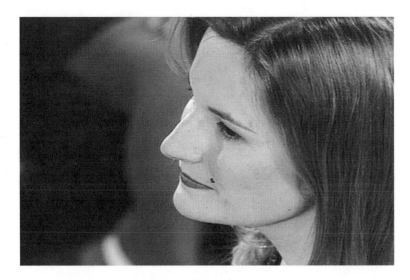

situated above the upper lip in the rhomboid area extending from the edge of the wing of the nose to the outer limit of the lip. This is an anatomical area named by comparative anthropologists as the "Cindy Crawford zone." By convention, localized deposits of melanin in this area are regarded as extremely attractive.

Now, in order to create the demonstration, we had to perform a type of surgery that had never been done on public television before. Our resident televisual cosmetologist (previously known as the "TV makeup person") underwent specialized and prolonged training which occupied nearly 80 percent of her tea-break. At the end of it Omani could be considered a fully qualified transplant surgeon in the area of plastic beauty-spot translocation. Without the use of anesthetics, Omani carefully removed the plastic beauty spot from Lisa's upper lip and successfully implanted it on the end of Lisa's nose. The audience, carefully taught beforehand all about how to demonstrate empathic, supportive, caring, sensitive responses, howled

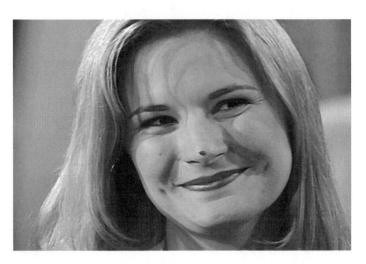

Skin: An Owner's Manual

with laughter. They couldn't help themselves. It's all to do with social expectations.

Beauty spots on the upper lip are gorgeous. Displaced to the tip of the nose they are regarded as risible. But of course this is simply a matter of convention. There is no reason whatever why it has to be that way. It would be easy to imagine a society that evolved on a small island in the South Seas where they simply decided that a beauty spot on the tip of the nose was stunningly attractive and to die for. If Cindy Crawford happened to visit there, they might find her quite repugnant.

Our culture is of course the other way around. We have depicted witches and hags as having spots on the ends of their noses in stories and illustrations for centuries. That pattern has been so deeply ingrained in our culture over the last dozen centuries or so that we cannot even imagine any other way of thinking about things. Which is why our studio audience laughed after the beauty-spot transplant—they couldn't do anything else.

This is an important point about our perceptions of beauty and ugliness. Even though it's difficult to accept as a fact, actually there is nothing intrinsically special or significant about these particular areas of the face. It is simply that as a culture we have decided to endow them with certain esthetic meanings. A daub of color *here* means beauty; the same daub of color *there* means ugliness. Yet these values are so deeply ingrained that it is almost impossible to imagine any other system of values. Try closing your eyes for a moment and thinking of a picture of, let's say,

Marilyn Monroe. Now try to imagine a society that could regard Marilyn Monroe as ugly or even repulsive. It's almost impossible, isn't it? The differences are miniscule, yet they are differences in which we have invested a great deal of significance. Beauty may be only skin deep, but since skin is almost all we see of other people, it's also true to say that beauty is only skin.

4

The Young and the Rashless

Now that we've discussed the basic structure and function of skin, let's move on to think about the way skin changes throughout the life of its owner and occupant.

For these purposes, we'll have a quick look at the skin problems specific to three ages or stages of human life: early in life, the teenage years, and maturity.

Truth Is Stranger Than Friction

Many years ago I did a TV studio demonstration using a rather neat machine which measured the smoothness of things. The design of that particular friction-meter was that it had a flat spinning wheel which you applied gently to the surface you were interested in. The machine measured the resistance to spin presented by the surface—very smooth surfaces offered very little resistance.

For the purposes of the demonstration, a young mother brought her six-month-old baby along to the studio and we diplomatically lowered the diaper and measured the smoothness of the baby's bottom. And the proverb was right—the skin of a baby's bottom is one of the smoothest biological substances in nature. This is probably because there is a great deal of subcutaneous fat, which is what makes the baby skin look so plump (and is probably a very useful survival feature, just in case there is a famine of some sort in the early days of the baby's life). Also the skin has got lots of elastic tissue in it (a very high amount in proportion to the other types of tissue), so it is basically wrinkle-free.

All of that is easy to understand, and makes intuitive sense. What may be a bit more surprising is that a baby's skin is actually pretty tough, despite its smoothness.

Red As a Baby's Bottom

When we think of a baby's bottom (and the manufacturers of diapers want us to do that as often as possible) we tend to think of something incredibly fragile and easily damaged.

Well, that's only true in certain ways.

If you observe a case of diaper rash, your first reaction is probably a heartfelt feeling of sympathy for the baby, and rightly so, because this rash is hugely uncomfortable for the baby. But your second reaction is that baby skin is incredibly fragile and ready at any moment to get inflamed and sore if it's allowed to get wet and stay wet. Which is only partially true.

In fact, a baby's bottom probably does benefit from being dry, but being simply wet is not such a major problem for medium periods of time. What causes diaper rash is actually a chemical irritation. The culprit is a chemical called ammonia. Ammonia is the same chemical that we smell in those household cleansing agents that are labeled "Contains Ammonia"—you know, it's the stuff that makes your eyes water. Anyway, ammonia can be produced from urine if it lies around and if there are the right sort of bacteria in the diaper area to do the production.

Finally, there is one other aspect of young skin that we can only guess at for the moment. It heals almost instantly after minor injures. Probably, like most tissues in babies and young people, the skin has a vast capacity to produce growth factors when challenged. This capacity diminishes in almost all tissues as we get old, and one of the most visible signs of aging (and I speak from personal experience here) is how long your skin takes to recover from minor injury. Even when you were a teenager a minor scrape or a cut would disappear in two or three days. In toddlers, tiny skin abrasions almost seem to disappear before your get the bandage out of the packet. It's very nice—and it's probably attributable to growth factors.

Speaking of growth, there are certain things that grow and flourish in skin at a later stage of our development which are completely and totally unwelcome and unwanted. We call them zits, so let's turn the page and talk about them next.

5

Thoroughly unfair Acne

Acne most commonly starts during puberty, which is extremely unfair of it.

As a friend of mine once put it, "By the time I was forty years old, I'd become pretty confident and socially buoyant. If only my acne had waited till then, I could have coped with it quite well. When I was fifteen it knocked me sideways."

That is the problem with puberty in general and acne in particular—it is a tidal wave of drastic and awkward changes that arrives at a very awkward time. And, of all these changes, the changes in the skin are the most visible and the most embarrassing and the unfair. So let's discuss what causes acne—and let me say immediately that acne is not caused by chocolate or anything you eat, and it's not caused by not washing or by anything else that you do or don't do. (With one exception: If you work in an oily atmosphere—such as in a kitchen frying food—and get droplets of oil on your face, or if you put a lot of oil on your hair and some drips onto your face, that can trigger acne. But eating or drinking the oil won't!)

There, I thought I'd get that message across right away. Now we can go back to the beginning and discuss what *does* cause acne and how it can be treated.

The "Spotted and Inconstant Youth"

The root cause of acne is...the root.

Well, actually it's in the sebaceous gland around the base of the hair root.

As you may remember from Chapter One, the sebaceous glands are the manufacturing plants for the oily lubricant sebum. As I said, sebum is probably an important component in the lubrication and waterproofing of skin. We think that there are sebaceous glands around each hair root because they are important in squirting sebum onto the hair as it grows out, which makes the entire animal more waterproof.

So as you can see in this picture, every hair-root has got at least one sebaceous gland built into the follicle (the socket where the root of the hair grows). The cells lining the sebaceous gland produce sebum,

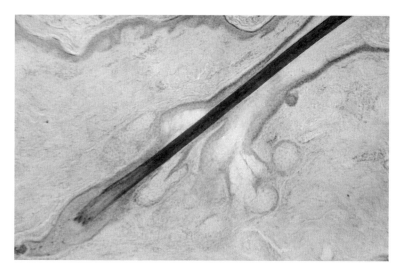

Hair-root and
sebaceous gland

which makes its way out of the gland via the thin duct of the gland.

Acne is caused by two factors: first, the amount of sebum produced by the sebaceous glands increases during puberty, and second, the ducts of the sebaceous glands become blocked FROM THE INSIDE.

Let's look at the increased production of sebum. It turns out that sebum production is increased under the influence of certain hormones and by far the most important of these is the male sex hormone, **testosterone**. As puberty gets going, there is a surge in testosterone level which produces (among all the other fascinating and eagerly awaited effects) a great increase in the production of sebum. Furthermore, the sebum probably becomes more oily and sticky at the same time. This might have been particularly useful at some stage in the evolution of the mammals. For example, a good volume of thick, sticky sebum might be just wonderful if you happen to be a beaver ready to go swimming around your underwater dam or something, but it is not all that helpful if you are a teenager getting ready for an important date on Saturday.

But that's only part of the problem. We could probably cope with an increase in sebum production, and probably even cope with an increase in viscosity (even on a Saturday) if the ducts of the sebaceous glands were willing and active participants in coping with the increased workload.

Unfortunately, although they do participate, it is entirely in the wrong way. They behave a bit like rubberneckers driving along in the traffic jam at an accident on the highway—they see a problem and are so keen to see more that they add to the problem. The traffic jam is mostly caused by people trying to see more of what is causing the traffic jam.

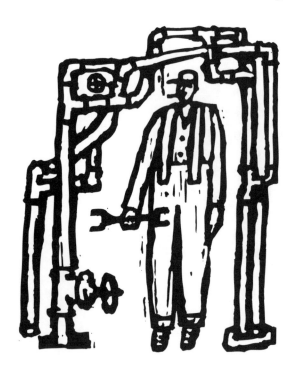

The cells lining the thin ducts of the sebaceous glands are a bit like that. They get over-enthusiastic (or so it seems—this is still a bit controversial) and they grow and multiply. This thickens the lining of the duct and thereby reduces the effective diameter of the duct. It's something like the way hard water furs up your water pipes—as the scale accumulates inside the pipe, the actual diameter of the hole in the middle for the water to go through is reduced. (I suppose it's lucky that our hot-water systems don't go through a puberty of their own; if they did we'd be in real trouble. Though what the furnace equivalent of acne would be nobody knows.)

Anyway, the net result of this combination of problems is that the sebaceous gland can't unload its sebum and so it gets distended and blown up with an accumulation of sebum. Eventually the distended sebaceous gland is big enough to make a small visible bump at the surface, which is colloquially known as a whitehead (medically known as a **comedo**, to prevent the patient from understanding anything about it).

So the whitehead is what you see when the duct is blocked and sebum accumulates behind it. Whiteheads are very common because the blockage in the duct usually happens at a point that is quite deep in the skin and not close to the surface. Sometimes, however, the blockage is nearer to the surface of the skin, and when that happens the normal bacteria that live on the skin surface—on everyone's skin surface, let me stress—can get into the accumulated oil and cause some changes.

When the normal skin bacteria—the ones that are happily camping on my skin at this moment—get into the oil, they change it. The first thing they do is to change the color of the oil: they make the sebum darker. In fact, the altered sebum looks dark brown or black, and this makes what we call a **blackhead**. Let me say absolutely clearly that a blackhead is produced when the sebum changes color. it is not caused by dirt! (In fact, it's likely to be made worse by scrubbing!)

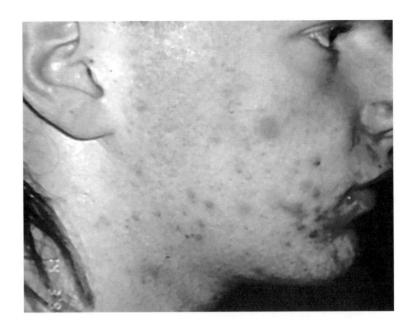

The normal bacteria also make the sebum become more acid, and a bit more of an irritant to the surrounding skin. The problems get worse from this point on. It's worth realizing that at this point the redness of a zit is due mostly to irritation of the surrounding skin because of the chemical effects of the sebum—it's not actually due to infection.

Unfortunately, infection often follows. The drop of oil is quite a pleasant environment for bacteria that may be lurking around below the surface of the skin and in the glands (who see it as we might see a huge buffet laid out on a nice table filled with all kinds of goodies).

What happens next is unfortunately predictable. The bacteria grow and the area of infection gets larger, with more inflammation around it. The infection results in the formation of pus. This is what we call a zit, the universally recognized word for something that medics insist on calling a **pustule** (to confuse the patients and make it sound as if the doctors are talking about something quite different).

In really severe cases, the facial skin can look like the photo of the young man on page 62. As we'll see in a moment, acne this bad is now treatable and nobody should have to suffer anything as bad as this nowadays.

Eventually (if the zit is left alone) the skin over the top of the pimple will break down and the infected material will discharge or drain into the outside world. That's what happens to most pustules—the discharge or draining process is the end of that particular zit. But unfortunately some pustules don't go away.

In some cases the pus doesn't drain away. The body's white blood cells go into action and move into the pus and kill the bacteria, but the fluid doesn't discharge into the outside world, it just stays there. What happens then is that the pus changes into a clear straw-colored liquid. A pimple where the pus has changed into this clear fluid is called a **cyst**. A cyst is a problem for two reasons. First, it might be quite big and it might look bad—cysts are usually very prominent and very visible. Second, a cyst is likely to heal with the formation of a scar.

What happens is that the body's emergency fix-it crews—including a group of particularly tough and hardy cells called the fibroblasts—move in when the usual self-renewing repair mechanisms can't get the job done. The fibroblasts lay down a little tough and light-colored strip of what we medics call fibrous tissue, which everyone else calls a scar. Usually the scar tissue occupies less space than the normal skin would have occupied, and certainly less space than the cyst did, so the surface of the skin looks pitted. These are the worst permanent consequences of acne, so avoiding scars is really important. Which means that acne that is very severe and is making cysts should be treated (as I'll explain in a moment).

What Makes Acne Worse

Now, before we go on to talk about the treatment of acne, it is perhaps worth spending a minute talking about a few things that can make acne worse—and the things that don't make acne worse (despite what busy-bodies tell you all the time).

In fact, let's start with the things that don't make acne worse. Here's a partial list:

- **Diet.** There is **no** relationship be-
  tween acne and anything you eat.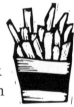
  That's right. Eating oily foods, french
  fries, chocolate, salad dressing, milk
  shakes—**none** of these affect acne in
  the slightest way.

- **Constipation.** No effect. You can be so consti-
  pated that going to the toilet makes your eyes water (which is medically a bad thing in itself) but
  constipation will not affect your acne. It might

cause problems for your hemorrhoids, your plumbing, your family members in line for the bathroom, but not for your acne.

- **Inefficient washing.** As I've explained, acne starts way below the surface of the skin. To blame it on inefficient washing is like blaming a delay in the subway system on inefficient street-cleaning in the road above the subway station.

- **New Age phenomena.** While we're on the subject, your acne will not be affected by the millennium (Y2K bugs don't live on the skin), the conjunction of the planets Venus and Mercury, the Dow-Jones, bad feng-shui, good feng-shui, whale-hunting, failing to rewind a rented video, or not putting the top back on the toothpaste.

There now, let's get on with some of the things that do have an effect.

- **Hormones.** As I said, the male sex hormone testosterone is a very powerful stimulator of skin changes that make acne more likely. Similarly, one of the female sex-hormones, **progesterone**, has the same effect. This is important because certain birth control pills have lots of progesterone, and if you are a woman on one of these, it's worth asking your doctor about if your acne is becoming a major problem.

On the other hand, another female sex hormone, **estrogen**, actually makes acne *better.* Since estrogen is also used in some birth control pills, the ones that have more estrogen and less progesterone may actually help.

- **Sweating.** Areas of the skin that sweat more profusely than average have a higher chance of developing acne. So, you may see more acne under your headband, for example, or under your bra.

- **Tropical weather.** By the same token, really hot and humid weather—we're talking genuine tropics here—may make acne worse. In fact, in the tropics acne is more common and often more severe.

- **Some (only a few) medications.** It's quite rare, but a few medications can make acne worse. If your acne does get worse after you've started a new medication, it's worth asking your doctor whether this is a recognized side-effect.

- **Stress.** Finally, most dermatologists agree that stress can make acne worse. And, of course, one of the greatest stresses in puberty is worrying about acne—and it's really unfair that the worrying by itself increases the chance of developing acne. It's also unfair that we live in a society that happens to revere perfect skin and teeth (not that anyone ever gets acne on their teeth, but you know what I mean). So before we get on the treatment of acne, let's talk for a moment about the social significance of acne.

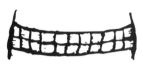

Zits of Passage

Incidentally, while we are talking about acne at the time of puberty (although, of course, acne can start at almost any age—people in their thirties and forties are by no means immune) the way we think about acne is rather peculiar. When we see a young man with the beginnings of a mustache or a beard we say to ourselves, "There's a boy turning into a man." A beard or a mustache is a rite of passage—it's a signal. We don't say to ourselves, "Yecch! There's a boy with hairs sticking out of his lip and chin." Yet although acne is a similar rite of passage, we never think of it like that. Nobody ever says, "Wow! He's sure growing into a wonderful hunk of a man—those biceps, that beard, that acne!"

Why?

Well, the answer is probably that humans seem to be hard-wired to avoid certain kinds of things. It seems likely that every animal species is programmed to avoid things that might be dangerous. For example, rotting meat. It would be a very considerable survival advantage for an animal to avoid anything that is actually decomposing, since a serious bacterial infection (or even death) might result. Hence the avoidance-reflex would flourish as an inherited trait. Probably human disgust with other things—vomit, feces, and so on—is linked to the same type of reflex. (Steven Pinker talks about this in some detail in his book *How the Mind Works*. People won't drink a soft drink if it has been stirred with a plastic mock-up of a piece of vomit, even if the toy has been taken out of its wrapper in front of them so they can see it's not the real thing.) Perhaps the sight of something that looks like pus triggers the same sort of reflex. Hence, I suggest, we come by our instinctive negative reaction to acne. It may just be a matter of inbuilt responses, although the response of other people to your acne can be quite dramatic.

Some studies show that people who have particularly bad acne suffer quite serious consequences in their social life and in the job-market. There are some studies which show that bad acne can reduce your chance of getting a job after an interview, which demonstrates the power of social signals sent out by the skin.

Of course, knowing all this doesn't make it any easier on the poor adolescent—but it does, perhaps, make it more logical to get bad acne treated so as not to suffer any of the visible after-effects.

Which brings us to the ways in which acne can be treated.

Death of the Zit—The Scarlet Pimple's Knell

The proper approach to the treatment of acne really depends on how bad the acne is, so let's divide the treatments into four main groups.

Mild Acne. The best approach is simply soap and water. Of course, soap and water won't stop the whiteheads forming—that happens well below the surface of the skin. But soap and water do reduce the number of bacteria on the skin, and so reduce the chance of large numbers of bacteria getting into the whiteheads and turning the color of the sebum darker. There is some evidence—not conclusive!—that those very lightly abrasive buffing pads may also help.

Mild to Moderate Acne. The message here is that one chemical is actually helpful. Its name is **benzoyl peroxide** and it happens to be an ingredient in most acne lotions. The other ingredients are a matter of personal taste and expense. If you happen to enjoy the feeling you get when using one particular lotion, go right ahead. But don't worry about the actual effect on your acne. As long as your lotion has got benzoyl peroxide in it, the cheap ones are just as good as the expensive ones.

Moderate to Severe Acne. Sometimes a pustule gets worse and worse. For those situations, it may be effective to use an antibiotic lotion—a lotion that contains an antibiotic. These are usually available only by prescription, but can be very helpful. The most commonly used antibiotics include things such as clindamycin, erythromycin, and a variety of others.

Another group of medications that work are a group of chemicals that resemble Vitamin A. These are called the **retinoids** and they have some useful effects on skin. For reasons that are not entirely understood (or at least not entirely understood by me), lotions that contain retinoids can be very helpful in treating bad acne. The most commonly used is **isotretinon** (Acutaine) which must NEVER be used in pregnancy. A new family of these medications called the **arotinoids** are being evaluated.

Severe Acne. If the acne is really bad—and particularly if cysts and scars are happening—then you may need treatment to be taken by mouth. There are two approaches here: antibiotics and retinoids. Taking antibiotics by mouth gradually changes the type of bacteria that live on the skin and alters the way they can mess about with the sebum. The important thing is to take the antibiotics exactly as prescribed, every day, for several months at least. Don't miss out a day here and there, and don't stop suddenly. The antibiotics used are usually the tetracyclines (including minocycline, for instance), but your doctor will tell you all about the one that she or he recommends.

In some cases your doctor may recommend retinoids by mouth instead of antibiotics. Again, it's very important to get the details right and take the medications exactly as prescribed.

Finally, we can spend a moment discussing a method of treatment that every person with acne probably tries at some stage. It's a self-administered treatment called squeezing.

Bringing Matters to a Head—To Squeeze or Not to Squeeze

The million dollar question which is one every teenager's lips (and chin, now that I come to think about it) is this: SHOULD ZITS BE SQUEEZED?

Well, there is an answer and the answer is—as a general rule—no. (Sorry, your mother was right on this one.)

On a few occasions, if—and it's a very important if—the zit is not infected and if it looks as though the plug in the follicle might be dislodged easily, then it's (probably) OK to give it just a gentle nudge. But if you do that, then just provide the ripe zit with something like a *hint* rather than a major high-pressure pincer-movement squeeze. If you do the gentle-nudging thing, and so help it to unplug itself the night before that important date or prom, you're probably all right. Giving a major squeeze to a deep-seated pimple that does not have an obvious (and loose) plug will probably allow the acid sebum to spread into the subcutaneous tissues around the hair follicle and increase the area of inflammation and redness. In other words, the visibility of the zit will be increased, and you'll be even more embarrassed on Saturday.

The Bottom Line

The basic message is a simple one, and an important one—bad acne is not something that "you simply have to put up with." Nobody nowadays should suffer really bad acne and the scars that follow it. So if your acne has gone past the mild or moderate stage, get some advice—it's really worth it.

6

Older Skin

Why We Need Clothes When We're Older

A traditional and doubtless apocryphal story has it that an antique dowager duchess drank far too much champagne at her eightieth birthday party, got into a wild and crazy mood, ripped off all her clothes, and streaked naked through the ballroom. One of her contemporaries, who had failing eyesight, peered at the nude pink behemoth and turned in astonishment to an equally elderly chap standing next to him and said, "That was Lady Elizabeth that just ran through the hall, wasn't it? And did you see what she was wearing?" To which his similarly short-sighted pal replied, "No, I didn't—but whatever it was, it needed ironing."

Such is the ultimate fate of all human skin—wrinkles. In the end, if we live long enough, we're all going to look as if we need ironing. It is undoubtedly true that *sic transit gloria mundi* (roughly translated that means "the glories of the world eventually disappear"). However, it is far more true, and far more important from the cosmetic viewpoint, that, before they disappear, most worldly glories go through a phase of either sagging or wrinkling. Some of them do both.

As it gets older, skin, by and large, seems to become too large for its owner-occupant. It no longer fits snugly. It wrinkles.

There are many factors which contribute to that. First of all, there is the loss of our childhood subcutaneous fat which, when we were young babies and totally adorable, made us all look so cuddly and plump and sweet.

When babies are born they have a lot of fat under the skin. This is important metabolically (or so it is thought) in that it protests the little fledgling against starvation in the first few days of life. So the miniscule incipient person arrives in the world with a nice little buffer of fat reserves under the skin. Furthermore, at the beginning of its life the baby's body has very little in the way of muscle tissue. Muscles develop in response to exercise, which is actually a very efficient and space-saving way of packaging the pre-adult form.

The infant contains the seeds (as it were) of muscles, which take up much less space than the final product will. So because of the plentiful fat and minimal musculature, the baby appears chubby and rounded and plump which we adore—and for a very good reason.

Human beings, like all advanced animal life forms, are pre-programmed to adore their offspring. This is a very important survival feature for every species—they must be particularly attracted to (and protective of) their children in order to further the continued survival of the species. When we see a little humanoid that's chubby and round and plump, we are hard-wired to say, "Oooohhh! How sweet!" (Of course, we manage to ignore the fact that it is also bald, has no teeth, and pees anywhere, all of which are characteristics we do not like half as much when we encounter them in late adulthood or old age.)

So because babies are plump and round and have soft skin, we have evolved (appropriately) the behavioral reflexes to become gooey whenever we see plump round soft-skinned things (including babies, peaches, kittens, Ewoks, buttocks, etc.) Which is fine for the babies. They just lie there being plump and round and we love them. But it has a down side: as human skin becomes older and looks less round and plump, we like it less.

As skin ages, it loses its plumpness by various methods. First, as we mature, much of our subcutaneous fat disappears and we begin to develop muscles. Hence as a young adult, the human being (particularly the male) begins to look much more angular and rippling. The female looks less angular than the male (in general) but is still much more angular than the baby. Which is all as it should be.

The problems begin in late adulthood. The skin loses its subcutaneous cushion of fat, and also the muscles that it covers begin to atrophy and shrink. Not only do those two things happen, but the skin also gets thinner—there is less of it. Even more significantly, as it thins it also begins to lose some specialized cells called **elastic fibers**. Let me explain.

The body's connective tissues come in a variety of types. There is the general "wrapping and foundation" type called **fibrous tissue**. There is also of course the fat, which is known medically as "fatty tissue" or **adipose tissue** if we think we're being overheard. Then there is a specialized variant of fibrous tissue called elastic tissue which contains specific fibers can be stretched but tend to return to their original length. Elastic tissue is very important in many areas of the body, notably in the lining of blood vessels, in the springy bit of the external ear, in the uterus, and in many other areas, including the skin.

The advantages of elasticity are obvious. It's the elasticity of the skin that gives it its shrink-fit, contour-hugging properties. The only snag is the elastic tissue just happens to wear out once you get into your late fifties or so. This loss of elastic tissue is what you can see for yourself in the test called the "elastic recoil test."

All you need to do it to take a gentle pinch of skin between finger and thumb and raise it a quarter or a half of an inch above the surface in a little ridge. Then

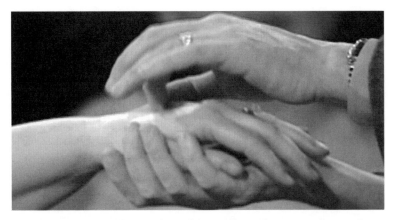

let go of the ridge. The skin ridge disappears in less than two seconds. In fact, in the younger person it's almost instantaneous. Once you are into your fifties and sixties the recoil is much slower, and in your later seventies it may take six or seven seconds before the ridge completely flattens out.

Sun, Sea, Sand, Smoke, and That Other Thing Beginning with S

The mechanisms that we've just been discussing—loss of subcutaneous fat, thinning of the skin itself, wasting of muscle tissue, and loss of elastic recoil—are the normal processes of aging that make skin liable to wrinkle. But in addition to the aging processes, there are things that we can do to our skin that make wrinkles appear in greater numbers and more quickly. Those things are the famous Five Ss. They are Sun (possibly with Sea and Sand), Smoke, and Smiles. (For those of you who thought that the Five Ss should include sex, I'm glad to tell you that sex doesn't actually causes wrinkles. It causes almost everything else you can think of—and a few things you can't—but not wrinkles).

Some things that cause wrinkles can be avoided—and some shouldn't be.

It is widely accepted that skin reacts to usage by wrinkling. Hence laughter-lines and frown-lines. While it is theoretically possible to reduce the eventual depth of these lines by avoiding facial expressions, this is not to be recommended (unless you make your living playing poker).

There is a popular move in certain high-profile strata of society to have some muscles of the face—the forehead, for example—paralyzed by special injections so that the muscles won't move and the skin won't wrinkle.

To me this seems as sensible as covering your new couch with a thick plastic cover so it won't get dusty. It may prolong that "newly-bought" appearance but it ruins the whole thing. You may have eternal youth as regards as your forehead, but in my opinion you end up looking a waxwork. Of course there are some people who would probably be better off—and do less damage to the world—if they could be miraculously turned into waxwork models, but that's a separate issue.

To put it simply, a few usage lines are what make a face look like a face. What we need is a little self-esteem and a little self-confidence. An obsession with preservation for its own sake produces an rather unhealthy appearance-fixated personality. As one writer put it so well: "When will the people who are incessantly worried about their reputation realize that that *is* their reputation?" The same is true of your facial appearance. If you are obsessed with your appearance, you seem to other people to be the kind of person who is obsessed with your own facial appearance and nothing else shows.

So, smile (and occasionally frown)—it proves you're not a waxwork.

Health Warning: Too Much Weather Is Not Good for Your Skin

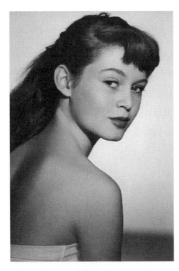

Young Bardot.

A few things look really good after the weather has beaten them for a few years (a copper roof, for example, looks far more noble after its tenth birthday), but skin doesn't.

What happens to skin after it has been exposed to lots of sun (and probably sea and wind) is that it becomes coarsened. It wrinkles much more easily.

Here's a fairly good example. This photograph is of a young woman whom I always thought would do well in the movies. Her name is Brigitte Bardot. She is a major fan of the beach and spends much of her time in the sun on the sand. Furthermore, she has always been a very public smoker of cigarettes. If you combine the sun, the sea, and the cigarette smoke, this is what happens to your skin: Basically, the skin loses even more of its elasticity than it nor-

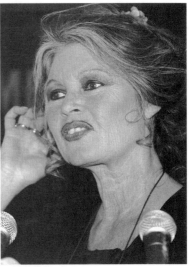

Bardot nowadays

mally would, it becomes incredibly wrinkled and puckered, and turns a sienna brown. In fact you basically end up looking like a leather purse with eyes.

So here's some advice. Take it easy with the suntan. Aside from the fact that actually burning the skin (i.e. a sunburn as opposed to a suntan) increases the risk of melanoma (see page 46), chronic exposure to sun gives you wrinkles. Or as we shall probably say in the future "it causes Bardotization of the skin."

Cigarette smoke makes it worse, probably due to the tars in cigarette smoke (rather than the nicotine, which is dangerous to most organs except the skin). So if you absolutely must smoke cigarettes, then put a paper bag over your head first, with a little hole to smoke the cigarette through. It may cause some odd looks at parties and dinners, but if you keep the bag over your head for the whole evening, nobody'll know who you are anyway.

Premature Aging of the Skin—A rare photo of the movie actress Monique de la Lala aged eighteen years. (Best known for her many appearances in the original *Star Trek* TV series in which she played the part of a rock on the planet Bjonka.)

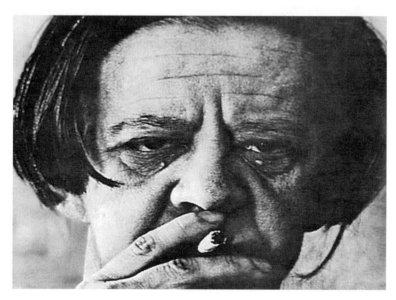

Wrinkles—What Can Be Done?

So, apart from avoiding too much sun, sea, and smoke, what can be done?

There is, of course, no total answer. There is nothing that will totally banish or prevent wrinkles, although every cosmetic and face cream manufacturer would love you to think otherwise.

There are, however, a few things that help a little bit.

The Alpha-Hydroxy Acids

There is a group of relatively simple acids, most of them found in fruit juices or similar sources, which happen to share a certain chemical structure. There are called the alpha-hydroxy acids. When applied to the skin in a relatively high concentration, they cause the top few layers of the skin to peel. This chemical peel has the cosmetic effect of taking the top layers of the wrinkle-ridges off, which makes the wrinkles appear shallower and the very shallow ones to disappear for a short time.

Hence a proper—and professionally supervised—chemical peel using alpha-hydroxy acids will give you a very slight and temporary improvement in your wrinkles.

Lower concentrations of alpha-hydroxy acids added to cosmetic products do not have any significant demonstrable effect.

Retinoids

As I mentioned in the previous chapter, the retinoids are a group of compounds that chemically resemble Vitamin A. For reasons that are not completely understood (yet) the retinoids, when applied to the skin, do have a mild but real effect in reducing wrinkles. It's really worth getting good advice on this, though, and it's also important to read the directions on the package carefully.

Vitamin E

We are only just beginning to understand Vitamin E. It's one of the vitamins that is soluble in fat (as opposed to the ones like Vitamin C that are soluble in water). When I was medical student, nobody knew what Vitamin E did. The only thing that was known about it was that if laboratory rats were totally deprived of Vitamin E they became sterile (i.e., infertile). This piece of knowledge seems to be of very limited importance unless you happened to be running an infertility clinic and most of your customers were laboratory rats.

In recent years, however, some very important features of Vitamin E have been discovered. It seems to have a useful effect on elastic tissue. For example, taken by mouth, Vitamin E seems to reduce the irritability of some important arteries and reduces their tendency to go into spasm and close down. This may be of great importance in the arteries that supply the heart muscle with blood—the coronary arteries. We've known for decades that the accumulation of sludge in the coronary arteries—atherosclerosis—is a major cause of heart attacks and angina.

But it seems that the sludge is not the only factor. In some people the coronary arteries seem to go into spasm easily, and they can make themselves very narrow without much provocation. In other people, even though there's a lot of sludge in the arteries, the chance of spasm is much less, and so serious problems are rarer. There is now some evidence that Vitamin E is one of the substances that reduces the chance of coronary arteries going into spasm. This would fit with the findings from some (but not all) studies that Vitamin E reduces the chance of heart attacks and death.

This may be related to the slight benefit of Vitamin E cream on skin. It is possible that a relaxing effect on elastic tissue may reduce the depth and the prominence of wrinkles.

Of course, as was famously said in a movie, one way to avoid wrinkles is to die young, so in the grand scheme of things it is much more important to avoid heart problems than it is to avoid wrinkles. But it's nice to know that Vitamin E may have a role in both and that it isn't simple a fertility drug for laboratory rats.

And the Shinbone's Connected to ... the Dishwasher

Wrinkling is not the only problem that afflicts older skin.

As we get older—and I have to confront the fact that the adjective now applies to me, not merely to everybody else—our skin loses some its speed and efficiency in healing and recovering from scrapes and trauma.

It is quite likely (but not yet certain) that this is related to the chemical signals which prod cells into growing and multiplying. These growth factors are super-abundant in the fetus and the infant (well, they would have to be, wouldn't they?) and almost certainly they gradually fade out as we get older. Or, perhaps, we get older *because* some of our cells produce less growth factors and other cells don't respond to them.

Either way, the skin doesn't heal as quickly as it used to. Minor nicks and cuts which would disappear in a day or two when you were a kid take several days to heal as you get older.

In fact, there are some areas of the body where this is particularly important—notably the inner surface of your shins. If you put your hands palm downwards of your knees, your thumbs are pointing down towards the inner surface of our shins. If you run your fingers down that surface you'll realize that on the inner surface, the skin rests directly on top of your bone (it's actually the tibia or shinbone). On the outside of your shins, the skin is well padded from below by a whole lot of muscles, but on the inside surface there's nothing much between the skin and the bone.

This means that an injury with a sharp object is likely to do more damage on the inner surface. A common example is banging your shin on something like an open dishwasher door—it often produces a wedge-shaped or triangular cut. Because this rests so directly over bone, it's actually quite difficult for that bit of skin to "get comfortable" while it's healing. Healing of those triangular cuts in the elderly is often a long-term problem. So if you are getting older, and if you go get a triangular cut on your inner shin, make sure you get your doctor's advice. The inner surface of your shin may not be as visible as wrinkles on your face, but it can be more important from a medical point of view.

And ALWAYS make sure the dishwasher door is closed before you walk past.

7

Skin Signals

Two-Way Traffic

So far, we've been talking about skin as a pretty remarkable and adaptable barrier keeping the animal inside safe and comfortable and the outside world firmly outside.

But skin is not only a frontier, it's also an interface, and the most important commodity that needs to travel in both directions across that interface is information.

Obviously any animal that has no idea what is happening in the outside world is in imminent and serious danger. Imagine being totally deprived of sensory information, perhaps like a sixteenth century knight in full armor, only without even the eye-slits in the visor, or someone sealed into a mobile version of one of those 1970s isolation-meditation samadi tanks. At any instant you could fall into a deep hole, or drown, or bake and overheat in the sun, or be eaten by predators, or starve to death if you couldn't locate any prey of your own. Your situation would be absolutely hopeless.

To stay alive, you need to know what's going on around you. That is why the skin has a vast range and number of sensory receptors that pick up different types of information about the outside world, translate that information into electric signals, and send those signals via the nerves to the brain. We call them the five senses, but of course there are more than five. Specialized receptors in the skin (and in the tissues just below it) sense a whole range of different types of information. There are the familiar ones: sight, sound, taste, touch, and smell, but there are also sensors for temperature, pressure, pain, fine touch, position (of limbs, digits, etc.), and others. When you stop to think about it, the human skin can sense almost any significant environmental factor except the phases of the moon and the Dow-Jones.

In any event, this is the important inward information traffic which the animal needs to survive and which the skin is compelled to receive and transmit to the brain.

Skin Signals

But there is also traffic in the other direction, which can sometimes be almost as important. In other words, it is also important for an animal to transmit information to the outside world, particularly to members of the same species, about the animal inside the skin.

From a rather simplified evolutionary point of view this might be a great help for the survival of the species. For example, try to imagine a herd of animals wandering along, say, a savanna. If one of the animals happens to come across something that is dangerous, it would be helpful to let the other animals know. If, for example, a gazelle is struck down by a lion, it would be a great help if all the other gazelles in the neighborhood ran away. Fast.

Strangely enough, this is probably why many species react so strongly to the sight of their own color of blood on their own species' skin: it's an important survival-beneficial behavioral reflex. Blood on the skin is an emergency warning signal, which is probably why humans universally use red as a danger signal. The same sort of thing is probably true of the "tail-up" flash of white underneath a rabbit's tail.

These species-specific signals are also a kind of information that has to go through the medium of the skin. So let's divide those skin signals into two groups: signals that transmit information about what's going on that minute (the state that the occupant of the skin is in at that moment) and the more long-term information about the stage or age of the animal.

"This Is The State I'm In" Skin Signals

As we've already discussed, there are some changes in or on the skin which have acquired an important emergency signaling function. The sight of blood on skin is just such a one. Any animal seeing red blood on the skin of a member of the same species and interpreting it as a sign of major and severe danger would have a survival advantage over an animal who didn't have that reflex and wandered over to see what was going on and got killed by the lion. Other physiological reactions to stress or danger also have signaling power.

The Birth of the Blues
For example, if a warm-blooded animal is exposed to unusual cold it will go blue. What actually happens is that the circulation of blood through the skin is slowed down (part of the body's reflex to try and conserve heat by directing more blood towards the inside of the body and away from the skin). As the red oxygen-carrying hemoglobin wends its way through the blood vessels in the skin, the oxygen leaves the red blood cells and is taken up by the cells in the tissues, and carbon dioxide is taken up by the hemoglobin in-

stead. Hemoglobin that is full of carbon dioxide has a slightly bluish tinge which is accentuated by the natural tinge of the skin. So when circulation is slow and there is more carbon-dioxide-carrying hemoglobin, the blood looks bluish (the medical word for this phenomenon is cyanosis). This doesn't happen when the circulation through the skin is fast. When the body is hot, the blood circulating through the skin moves briskly, and the hemoglobin keeps its reddish tinge so the skin looks red and not blue. But in the cold, cyanosis of the skin happens.

Of course, an animal does not *decide* to go blue, but when it happens it means that the animal is coping with (or suffering from) cold and other members of the same species interpret that as an important signal, a statement about what the environment is like.

It'll Be All White on the Night

Paleness (the correct medical term is "pallor") of the skin is also a significant skin signal.

Basically, when an animal loses a lot of blood or goes into the medical condition known as shock (when the blood pressure falls to very low levels because of hemorrhage or infection), the body diverts blood to the areas that need it (the heart, brain, kidneys) and away from areas that are "luxuries" (the guts, genitals, and skin, for example). Hence in shock, the skin goes pale. Most animals—humans included—interpret sudden pallor of the skin of a fellow as a sign of something seriously amiss, so it, too, is a way in which the physiological state of the skin has signaling power.

The same involuntary reflex system can also be activated by psychological factors. Hence when someone sees or hears something that is deeply and suddenly upsetting, the same reflexes can be activated and the person turns pale. When we see someone turning pale we interpret that, quite correctly, as somebody being seriously shocked. Our interpretation is a refined and socialized product of a response to an important biological phenomenon.

Blushing

However, not all signals are emergency warnings like hemorrhage, cyanosis, or pallor. Some are quite nice. Blushing is an example of a "nice" signal.

Some people blush easily. In the TV studio, I made a volunteer blush very readily simply by asking her to "moon" the TV audience. She went bright red simply at the *thought* of mooning.

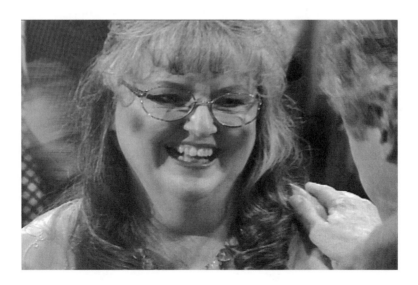

The origins of that reflex are interesting. Apparently, among the higher apes the blushing signal is a flush that covers the face, neck, and upper chest area of mature females. It is probably mediated by several hormones which include the female sex hormone estrogen. Hence, only sexually mature apes can blush. This means that the blush signal among apes indicates the mate-ability of the blusher. Had a male orangutan been present in the studio he would have found our volunteer's flush extremely attractive.

In humans, of course, blushing has evolved into a social signal of embarrassment, albeit far more prevalent in mature individuals and in women than in men.

So, if you blush excessively what can you do? The answer is, unfortunately, not very much. If you feel a blush coming on at a cocktail party or something, you can look around and see if there are any good-looking orangutans who have noticed it (there usually are), but otherwise the best way to cope is to acknowledge it. Like all factors which threaten a conversation or interaction, the effect is considerably diminished by acknowledgment. If you are able to make a comment about how you blush very easily and this is just one of those embarrassing moments, then the emotional ripples will stop spreading. You will (to some extent) get control of the situation and this will reduce the extent and the duration of the blush. And as always, a little bit of upbeat self-acknowledgment is an attractive feature in and of itself, whether it appeals to orangutans or not.

Sweating

In the same category as blushing is the emotional type of sweating. As we've already discussed, sweating is a useful physiological response to a warm or hot environment, but it also may be switched on under the influence of emotional states such as anxiety. In a few very rare cases, sweating from the armpits can be so profuse as to be a very serious social handicap.

This type of skin signal probably had (or has) some survival value. If you're in a tough spot, it probably helps to let other people know that.

For those few people who have a really serious and socially-disabling problem with sweating there are some measures that might be helpful. For a start, there are some extremely powerful anti-perspirants nowadays (such as Drysol) which are much more effective than their predecessors. For very unusual and severe cases, the sympathetic nerves to the armpit can be cut in a surgical operation, or part of the armpit skin can be surgically removed. Injections of botulinus toxin can also sometimes help.

"This Is The Stage I'm At" Signals

To some extent, all the changes that accompany the aging process are signals. Or, to be a little more accurate, human beings have learned to recognize the signals of aging in the skin.

As we saw earlier, humans regard human skin that is soft, plump, dimpled, and hairless—when it is on a small-sized humanoid form—as adorable, because it occurs on young babies and we are programmed to adore our babies. As the infant grows older, we recognize the loss of the roundness and plumpness as a sign of advancing maturity, and the subsequent appearance in males of facial hair (and sometimes acne) as a harbinger of imminent fathering (i.e., child-producing) potential. Yet there is another signaling system directly related to the hair which has extraordinary species-specific power, and that is the distribution of hair around the skin.

Gimme Hair

At the time of puberty, not only does the growth of hair change, but so does its distribution—where it flourishes. As we all know, at the time of puberty males grow hair on the face, under the armpits, on the limbs, and in the pubic area. What we all know but may not have realized as a conscious fact is that pubic hair has a gender-specific distribution. In females, the hair stops at a horizontal "bikini" line. In males the pubic hair has a diamond-shaped distribution, the bottom half of the diamond pointing downwards to the genitals, the top half pointing upwards to the navel.

Now, I'll try not to get all coy and bashful about this subject, nor to be too brazen or prurient, but let's think for a moment about the symbolic power of pubic hair. It is, after all, no more than hair—a little bit shorter and curlier than most of the other hairs on the person, but not vastly different in any other way. Yet even a glimpse of pubic hair is an intense erotic signal in a way with which (let's be honest) nostril hair or armpit hair cannot compete. If you think for a moment about how you would react to a view of three hairs from someone's armpit (think of a favorite film star for example) compared to three hairs from the same person's pubis, you will see the intense symbolic power of secondary sexual characteristics. And rightly so. After all, successful mating is essential to the survival of the species, so it is not surprising that symbols of sexual maturity have intense signaling power.

Involuntarily, our response to all the signals associated with successful mating are imbued with the power of the procreational urge. And it's that power which helps advertisers use sexual signals to sell every consumer product on this planet (including, so I'm told, sex).

It's a simple matter of using what the human species is designed to do naturally.

So far we've been discussing nature-made skin signals, but of course our entire species indulges in a wide range of human-made (i.e., artificially manufactured) skin signals which can be conveniently divided into two categories, temporary and permanent.

Temporary Artificial "Stage" Signals

The most important and widely-used skin signals that make up this category are called . . . makeup.

Humans, unlike any other animal species that I know of, enhance various anatomical features of their skin with artificial coloring. And it is very interesting to think about which features are decorated by makeup. Most of the areas that are highlighted are the parts of the skin where the ordinary type of skin meets the mucous membranes (such as the lining of the mouth and the eyes). It so happens that these areas—called the muco-cutaneous junctions—become highly sensitive during puberty and stay that way for decades. Most of the erogenous zones are muco-cutaneous junctions (though only a few—i.e., the lips—are socially acceptable zones for lipstick, of course). Other areas do receive cosmetic attention—the cheekbones earn blusher quite often—but in terms of priorities, most women would rather be seen wearing lipstick but no blusher rather than the other way round.

If you visited this planet from another part of the galaxy, you might be mystified as to why so many humans should use one of thirty thousand shades of a few colors to emphasize their lips and never use any color on, say, their ear-lobes and nostrils. Also, the colors 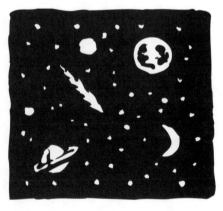 that are used are generally fairly close to blood-tones or flesh-tones—emerald-green lipstick or yellow-ochre would usually be regarded as highly deviant.

Similarly the eyelids are decorated with eyeshadow and eyeliner, but the rims of the nostril aren't. The fingernails and the toenails are routinely and carefully painted in the female, but the knuckles aren't. Nor are the tops of the ears. Presumably these rituals have evolved because these areas have a particularly important signaling function. In other words, our responses to nicely painted nails or delicately mascaraed eyelashes are part of our involuntary repertoire of human reflexes. We may think we're responding out of pure rational and esthetic choices, but we may actually be impelled by more (literally) animal forces.

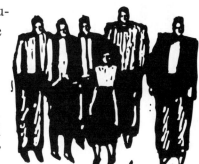

So when you watch a crowd of people around the cosmetics counter in a department store and think, "This is a zoo," you're probably right.

Permanent Artificial "Stage" Signals

There is a permanent and equally ritualized form of makeup which exists or has existed in almost every human race and that is the tattoo. (The modern politically correct term seems to be "skin art," although, personally, I always think that sounds like a polite term for striptease.)

Tattooing is the implanting of particles of dye deep in the skin near the basal layers, where they will not be brought up to the surface and scuffed off. That's why they are permanent. The social conventions surrounding tattoos would make the subject of a book in themselves (actually, they have, and this isn't it). Until recently, in North America and Europe it was a symbol of lower socio-economic status and was commonest among the armed forces. Often the tattoo would be in the form of a name. (Which always made me wonder. I mean, if a man tattoos "I Love Gladys" on his biceps and then breaks up with Gladys, what are his options? Will he be able to find a new girl-friend called Doris, let's say, who doesn't mind snuggling into Gladys's name on his arm at night? Or does he have to spend the rest of his life only going out with girls called Gladys? It's a dilemma, isn't it?) Anyway, nowadays, tattoos are very chic, with some overtones of being a bit risqué. They are quite common on female shoulders and ankles (which I personally have always regarded as quite significant erogenous zones of their own, actually).

What's really interesting about tattoos, though, is that in developing countries there are entire languages of tattoos. In various areas of Africa and the South Seas, the entire history of the individual may be expressed in tattoos—child-bearing history, status among other warriors, etc.

When you add up all these different ways in which skin can send powerful signals to other humans, it does make you realize how much you tell other people—and find out from them—without using any words.

No wonder kissing is such an important transaction.

8

More Sinned Against Than Sinning

This has been something of a helter-skelter, frenzied dash around human skin, and, as I said at the outset, I've only selected a few of what I regard as the most fascinating topics to discuss. I hope you've found some of them equally intriguing.

Your skin is the main way you have of making contact with the world and vice versa. It's the walls of your biological home and an integral part of everything that your home is and does for you. Apart from painting it, sunblocking it, and anti-wrinkling it, in our everyday life we usually ignore most of its biological functions (unless something goes wrong with it).

But our skin merits a bit more attention than that. It's the wrapper you came in and you can't discard it without destroying the contents. From the evolutionary and biological point of view, beauty is not simply skin deep, beauty is only skin.

So it's worth a bit of care, attention, and, above all, appreciation to keep it in good shape.

Acknowledgments

I had a lot of help from two wonderful dermatologists, friends and colleagues Dr. Neil Shear (who also read the entire manuscript), Professor and Dermatologist at the Sunnybrook Health Science Centre, University of Toronto, and Dr. Lynn From (who also provided the photomicrographs on pages 30 and 41), Professor and Dermatologist, Women's College Hospital, University of Toronto.

My executive assistant, supporter, and companion Susan Mawhood did the research for the illustrations. At PBS Detroit I had tireless cooperation from Diane Bliss, Jay Nelson, Marty Goodman, and Chris Benjamin, and at Lark International from Bill Nemtin and Chuck Rossi. At TV Books, my new colleague Keith Hollaman tolerated the fairly typical vagaries of a medical author with aplomb.

The factual details of this book were checked by a combination of the above people. As regards the explanations of biology and evolution, the many and varied hypotheses, and the jokes, I cannot find anyone to blame except myself.

Photographs on pages 10 (paramecium protozoan)

and 18 (hair root) Corbis/Lester V. Bergman; page 14 illustration by Martin Nichols, from *What You Really Need to Know about Cancer,* by Dr. Robert Buckman, courtesy of The Johns Hopkins University Press; page 26 (house dust mite) copyright 1999 Volker Steger/Peter Arnold, Inc.; pages 40 (Buckman's hand with Julia's), 49, 50, 77 (elastic recoil test), and 91 (blushing woman) courtesy of Detroit Public Television; pages 30 and 41 courtesy of Lynn From (photomicrographs of skins); pages 45 and 80 courtesy of the Canadian Cancer Society; page 62 courtesy Hoffman-LaRoche; page 79 (2 Bardot images) Corbis/Bettman.

Index

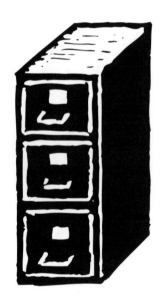

About the Author

D
R. ROBERT BUCKMAN is a professor in the Department of Medicine at the University of Toronto and an oncologist at the Toronto-Sunnybrook Regional Cancer Centre. For the past twenty years he has had a second career in communication and broadcasting, presenting television science-and-medicine programs in Britain and Canada. Two of his television series ("Don't Ask Me" and "Where There's Life") have aired on the Discovery Channel.

He has written ten books, including *What You Really Need to Know About Cancer* and *I Don't Know What to Say: How to Help and Support Someone Who is Dying*. He is currently working on a series of medical information videos with John Cleese as co-writer.

He is married to a gorgeous and tolerant Canadian physician who believed him when he said he had an immense personal fortune and a heart complaint. He is currently attempting to acquire one or the other.